My Innovative Dash Diet

Fit and Healthy Recipes for Your Everyday Meals

Eleonore Barlow

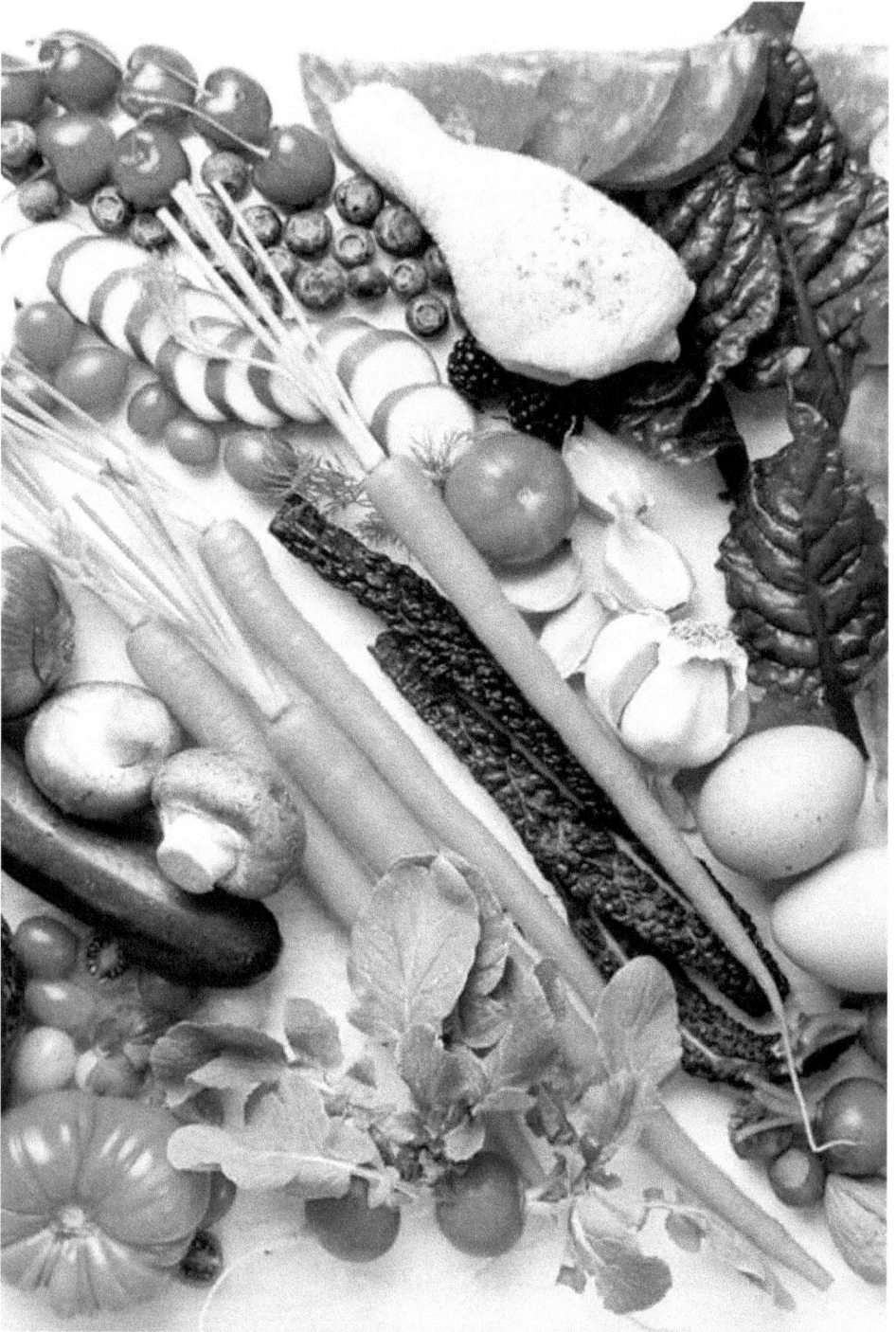

Table of Contents

Barley, Grape Tomato and Arugula Sauté

SmartPoints value: Green plan - 3SP, Blue plan - 3SP, Purple plan - 1SPTotal time: 50 min, Prep time: 10 min, Cooking time: 40 min, Serves: 4

Nutritional value: Calories - 82.8, Carbs - 4.8g Fat - 7.2g, Protein - 1.2g

This grain and vegetable side dish is colourful and sweet with a peppery bite.

Toss in some yellow grape tomatoes to add even more colour.

Ingredients

Water - 1¼ cup(s)

Table salt - ¾ tsp, divided

Pearl barley (uncooked) - ½ cup(s)

Olive oil (extra-virgin) - 1½ tsp, divided

Tomatoes (grape) - 1½ cup(s), halved

Minced garlic - 1½ tsp

Black pepper (freshly ground) - ¼ tsp

Arugula (baby leaves) - 3 cup(s)

Lemon zest (finely grated) - ¼ tsp (or to taste)

Instructions

1.   Stir half tsp of salt into a small saucepan of water and bring it to a boil. Add barley to it and cover; reduce the heat to low and cook until the water is absorbed and the barley is tender but still has a nice bite to it; about 30-35 minutes. Remove the saucepan from the heat and set it aside.

2.   Apply heat to one teaspoon of oil in a medium nonstick skillet over medium-high heat. Add the tomatoes and garlic, then sauté it until the tomatoes start to soften and release their juices; about 1-2 minutes.

3.   Put in more barley, the remaining one-quarter teaspoon of salt and

pepper, and reduce the heat to medium and cook, stirring it until the tomatoes soften further and the grain absorbs tomato liquid; about 2-3 minutes.

4.   Stir in the arugula and toss it over medium heat until it wilts; about 30 seconds.

5.   Remove the dish from the heat and stir in the remaining half teaspoon of oil and lemon zest.

Note: You can reheat this recipe the next day, and it will still taste great. Alternatively, you can serve it as a cold salad. Allow it come to room temperature and then toss it, adding just a bit of red wine or balsamic vinegar.

Creamy Mushroom and Chicken Stew Crockpot

SmartPoints value: Green plan - 2SP, Blue plan - 2SP, Purple plan - 2SP

Total Time: 4hr 20min, Prep time: 10 min, Cooking time: 4hr 10mins,

Serves: 4

Nutritional value: Calories – 278, Carbs – 24.2g, Fat – 4.2g, Protein – 32g

The mushroom and chicken stew crockpot is a fantastic low-calorie dinner idea. It's a healthy and easy slow cooker recipe with great taste.

Ingredients

Chicken breast (skinless) - 1 lb

Baby portabella mushroom (sliced) - 8 oz

Onion (finely chopped) - 1 piece

Carrots (cut into matchsticks) - 1/2 cup

Peas (fresh or frozen) - 1/2 cup

Celery (chopped) - 2 stalks

Mushroom seasoning (powdered) - 2 tbsp

Chicken broth (fat-free) - 2 cups

Sour cream (fat-free, at room temp) - 1 cup

Garlic (minced) - 3 cloves

Salt (1 tsp)

Pepper (1/2 tsp)

Instructions

1.   Combine all ingredients in a crockpot except the sour cream.

2.   For 4- 6 hrs., cook on low heat.

3.   For about 5 minutes, stir in sour cream, and warm until it is thoroughly heated. Serve immediately.

Smashed Avocado and Egg Toast

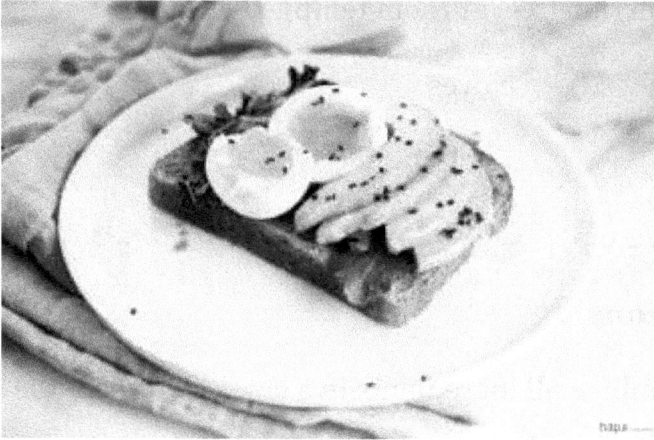

SmartPoints value: Green plan – 6SP, Blue plan – 4SP, Purple plan - 4SP

Total Time: 7 min, Prep time: 5 min, Cooking time: 2 min, Serves: 1

Nutritional value: Calories – 214.0, Carbs - 16.4g, Fat – 14.2g, Protein - 8.4g

Ingredients

Avocado - ¼ item(s), medium-sized, ripe but still a touch firm

Light whole-grain bread - 1 slice(s)

Whole hard-boiled egg(s) - 1 item(s), sliced

Table salt - 1 pinch

Crushed red pepper flakes - 1 pinch

Black pepper - 1 pinch

Instructions

1.   Place one slice of bread on a clean plate.

2.   Top with a portion of peeled avocado and gently smash with a knife or fork.

3.   Cut hard-boiled egg in half and place each half on the bread.

4.   Gently smash egg and mix with smashed avocado. Season the bread to taste with salt, pepper, and red pepper flakes.

5.   Cover with another slice of bread and place in a flat-sitting electric bread toaster.

6.   Remove smashed avocado and egg toast from the toaster once the "ready" light comes on.

Sweet Pineapple and Strawberry Salsa with Yogurt

The best salsas sometimes don't contain tomatoes, and this sweet pineapple and strawberry salsa with yogurt recipe is a good example.

I've added coconut flakes to this recipe to give a pleasant taste of fresh fruit.

SmartPoints value: Green plan – 3SP, Blue plan – 2SP, Purple plan - 2SP Total Time: 8 min, Prep time: 4 min, Cooking time: 4 min Serves: 1 Nutritional value: Calories - 30.9, Carbs - 7.4g, Fat - 0.4g, Protein - 0.4g

Ingredients

Strawberries - 3 medium-sized, diced - fresh mint leaves - 1 tsp (chopped)

Pineapple - ½ cup(s), Golden species (diced)

Plain fat-free Greek yogurt - ½ cup(s)

Lime zest - ⅛ tsp (grated)

Unsweetened coconut flakes - 1 Tbsp (toasted)

Coconut flakes – 3 Tbsp

Instructions

Dice strawberries, pineapple, mint, and lime zest into a small bowl, all mixed.

Add yogurt and speckle with coconut. You can also spoon the yogurt into a glass dish and top it with fruit and coconut.

Creamy Banana French Toast Casserole

You can give a bright flavor to this creamy casserole and also keep the banana from turning black by adding a small quantity of lemon juice.

SmartPoints value: Green plan – 7SP, Blue plan – 6SP, Purple plan - 6SP

Total Time: 55 min, Prep time: 20 min, Cooking time: 35 min, Serves: 12

Nutritional value:

Calories - 489, Carbs - 68.7g, Fat - 18g, Protein - 15.4g

Ingredients

Cooking spray - 5 spray(s)

Whole wheat/oatmeal bread - 12 slice(s), cut into quarters (about 1 oz per slice)

Neufchâtel cheese - 4 oz, (1/3-less-fat cream cheese)

2% reduced-fat milk - 1 cup(s)

Maple syrup - ½ cup(s)

Egg(s) - 6 large

Banana(s) - 4 medium-sized, ripe (divided)

Fresh lemon juice - 2 tsp

Rum - 1 Tbsp

Ground cinnamon - ½ tsp

Vanilla extract - 1 tsp

Ground nutmeg - ½ tsp

Table salt - ¼ tsp

Powdered sugar - 3 Tbsp

Instructions

1. Get a clean 13 inches by 9 inches baking dish and coat it with cooking spray.

2. Stand quarter portions of bread up in the prepared dish, so it lines the sides and bottom in a single layer — Preheat the oven to 350°F.

3. Place the cheese, milk, and syrup in a blender.

4. Add eggs, two bananas, rum, vanilla, juice, nutmeg, cinnamon, and salt to the blender.

5. Allow the blending process to Dash until the mixture is smooth.

6.   Gently pour the mixture over the bread and press those on the sides of the baking dish into the egg mixture, making sure it is completely submerged.

7.   Refrigerate the dish for 30 minutes after covering with foil.

8.   Preheat the oven again to 350°F. Just before baking, thinly slice the remaining two bananas and put the slices in between pieces of bread.

9.   Cover the dish with new foil and bake for 25 minutes. Remove the foil and continue baking until the color is golden brown. Set for about 10 minutes more, then sprinkle the top with powdered sugar. Slice the casserole into 12 pieces and serve immediately.

Note: You can serve with fresh berries if you desire.

Fried Egg with Asparagus-Potato Hash

Eggs look great with asparagus in this fantastic breakfast recipe. To effortlessly prepare asparagus so that the cooking will be fast and be tender, bend the spears near the tail until the woody part breaks off. You can also use the points of the spears and reserve the middle of the asparagus stalks for another preparation like a veggie stir-fry or steamed in a green salad. You should microwave the potato and then sauté it. Microwaving ensures that the interior is soft, with a crisped, browned exterior, a perfectly hashed topping to your egg.

SmartPoints value: Green plan – 7SP, Blue plan – 5SP, Purple plan - 1SP Total Time: 22 min, Prep time: 12 min, Cooking time: 10 min, Serves: 1 Nutritional value: Calories - 319, Carbs - 38.4g, Fat - 8g, Protein - 11.5g

Ingredients

Uncooked red potato(es) - 1 medium-sized, pierced severally with a fork

Uncooked asparagus - 4 spear(s), medium-sized, trimmed, diagonally sliced 1/2-inch thick (1/2 cup)

Uncooked scallion(s) - 1 small (sliced)

Olive oil - 1 tsp

Table salt - ¼ tsp

Fresh thyme - 1 tsp (chopped)

Egg(s) - 1 large, cooked sunny-side up

Black pepper - 1 pinch

Instructions

1. Microwave potato for about 3-4 minutes and cut into small dice.

2.   Heat the oil in a medium-sized, nonstick skillet over a medium to high heat.

3.   Add the asparagus and diced potato to the oil

4.   Cook, occasionally stirring, until the diced potatoes are browned, and asparagus is crisp-tender, about 4 minutes.

5.   Add the scallion and thyme; keep stirring until scallion wilts, about 30 seconds.

6.   Season with salt and pepper, then serve with egg.

Greek-Style Scrambled Eggs

If you need a quick and easy weeknight dish, you can prepare these scrambled eggs within 20 minutes. These eggs make a perfect one-dish meal, loaded with various flavors that include butter beans, chicken chorizo sausage, grape tomatoes, and onions.

To make this meal vegetarian, add soy-based breakfast sausage. You can use lentils in place of butter beans if you can't find them.

Prevent overcooking by turning off the heat before the eggs are all the way cooked.

SmartPoints value: Green plan – 8SP, Blue plan – 3SP, Purple plan - 3SP Total Time: 20 min, Prep time: 12 min, Cooking time: 8 min, Serves: 1 Nutritional value: Calories - 221, Carbs - 5.1g, Fat - 10.3g, Protein - 21.0g

Ingredients

Cooked chicken chorizo sausage - 1½ oz (diced)

Cooking spray - 5 spray(s)

Canned butter beans - ¼ cup(s), rinsed and drained

Crumbled feta cheese - 1 Tbsp

Uncooked onion(s) - ¼ cup(s) (chopped)

Grape tomatoes - 6 medium-sized (halved)

Egg(s) - 2 large

Black pepper - 1 pinch, or add to taste

Table salt - 1 pinch, or add to taste

Dill - 1 Tbsp, chopped

Instructions

1.   Coat a medium-sized nonstick skillet with nonstick spray.

2.   Add chicken chorizo and onion, then cook over medium heat, occasionally stirring, until lightly browned, about 5 minutes.

3.   Add tomatoes and beans, then stir until the tomatoes start to soften, about 1 minute.

4.   Push the mixture to one side of the skillet and add eggs to the other side.

5.   Scramble the eggs until softly set, 1-2 minutes.

6.   Turn in the chorizo mixture and season with salt and pepper, then sprinkle with dill and feta.

Black Bean Vegan Wraps

Nutritional Facts

servings per container	5
Prep Total	**10 min**
Serving Size 2/3 cup (27g)	
Amount per serving **Calories**	**200**
	% Daily Value
Total Fat 8g	**1%**
Saturated Fat 1g	2%
Trans Fat 0g	2%
Cholesterol	**2%**
Sodium 240mg	**7%**
Total Carbohydrate 12g	**2%**
Dietary Fiber 4g	14%
Total Sugar 12g	01.21%
Protein 3g	
Vitamin C 2mcg	2%
Calcium 20mg	1%
Iron 7mg	2%
Potassium 25mg	6%

Ingredients

1 1/2 half cup of beans (sprouted & cooked)

2 carrot

1 or 2 tomatoes

2 avocados

1 cob of corn

1 Kale

2 or 3 sticks of celery

2 persimmons

1 Coriander

Dressing:

1 hachiyapersimmon (or half a mango)

Juice of 1 lemon

2 to 3 tablespoons original olive oil

1/4 clean cup water

1 or 2 teaspoons grated fresh ginger

1/2 teaspoon of salt

Instructions:

1.   Sprout & cook the black beans

2.   Chop all the ingredients & mix them in a neat bowl with the black beans

3.   Mix all the ingredients for the dressing & pour into the salad

4.   Serve a spoonful in a clean lettuce leaf that you can easily roll into a wrap. Most people do use iceberg or romaine lettuce.

Fascinating Spinach and Beef Meatballs

Serving: 4

Prep Time: 10 minutes

Cook Time: 20

Ingredients:

½ cup onion

4 garlic cloves

1 whole egg

¼ teaspoon oregano

Pepper as needed

1-pound lean ground beef

10 ounces spinach

How To:

1.   Preheat your oven to 375 degrees F.
2.   Take a bowl and blend within the remainder of the ingredients, and using your hands, roll into meatballs.

3.   Transfer to a sheet tray and bake for 20 minutes.

4.   Enjoy!

Nutrition (Per Serving)

Calorie: 200
Fat: 8g
Carbohydrates: 5g
Protein: 29g

Juicy and Peppery Tenderloin

Serving: 4

Prep Time: 10 minutes

Cook Time: 20

Ingredients:

2 teaspoons sage, chopped

Sunflower seeds and pepper

2 1/2 pounds beef tenderloin

2 teaspoons thyme, chopped

2 garlic cloves, sliced

2 teaspoons rosemary, chopped

4 teaspoons olive oil

How To:

1.   Preheat your oven to 425 degrees F.

2.   Take alittle knife and cut incisions within the tenderloin; insert one slice of garlic into the incision.

3.   Rub meat with oil.

4.   Take a bowl and add sunflower seeds, sage, thyme, rosemary, pepper and blend well.

5.   Rub the spice mix over tenderloin.

6.   Put rubbed tenderloin into the roasting pan and bake for 10 minutes.

7.   Lower temperature to 350 degrees F and cook for 20 minutes more until an indoor thermometer reads 145 degrees F.

8.   Transfer tenderloin to a chopping board and let sit for 15 minutes; slice through 20 pieces and enjoy!

Nutrition (Per Serving)

Calorie: 183

Fat: 9g

Carbohydrates: 1g

Protein: 24g

Healthy Avocado Beef Patties

Serving: 2

Prep Time: 15 minutes

Cook Time: 10 minutes

Ingredients:

1 pound 85% lean ground beef

1 small avocado, pitted and peeled

Fresh ground black pepper as needed

How To:

1.   Pre-heat and prepare your broiler to high.

2.   Divide beef into two equal-sized patties.

3.   Season the patties with pepper accordingly.

4.   Broil the patties for five minutes per side.

5.   Transfer the patties to a platter.

6.   Slice avocado into strips and place them on top of the patties.

7.   Serve and enjoy!

Nutrition (Per Serving)

Calories: 568

Fat: 43g

Net Carbohydrates: 9g

Protein: 38g

Ravaging Beef Pot Roast

Serving: 4

Prep Time: 10 minutes

Cook Time: 75 minutes

Ingredients:

3 ½ pounds beef roast

4 ounces mushrooms, sliced

12 ounces beef stock

1-ounce onion soup mix

½ cup Italian dressing, low sodium, and low fat

How To:

1.   Take a bowl and add the stock, onion soup mix and Italian dressing.

2.   Stir.

3.   Put roast beef in pan.

4.   Add mushrooms, stock mix to the pan and canopy with foil.

5.   Preheat your oven to 300 degrees F.

6.   Bake for 1 hour and quarter-hour .

7.   Let the roast cool.

8.   Slice and serve.

9.   Enjoy with the gravy on top!

Nutrition (Per Serving)

Calories: 700

Fat: 56g

Carbohydrates: 10g

Protein: 70g

Rainbow Nourishment Bowl

Nutritional Facts

servings per container	5
Prep Total	**10 min**
Serving Size 2/3 cup (77g)	
Amount per serving **Calories**	**20**
	% Daily Value
Total Fat 2g	**0%**
Saturated Fat 7g	2%
Trans Fat 0g	10%
Cholesterol	**5%**
Sodium 55mg	**20%**
Total Carbohydrate 9g	**200%**
Dietary Fiber 7g	1%
Total Sugar 36g	2%
Protein 1g	
Vitamin C 6mcg	21%
Calcium 160mg	2%
Iron 7mg	2%
Potassium 320mg	10%

Ingredients

2 cups spinach

1/2 cup corn kernels

1/2 cup edamame beans

1/2 cup cabbage, shredded

1/4 cup carrots, sliced

1/2 cup quinoa, cooked

1 radish, sliced

Handful pea shoot sprouts (or another type of sprouts)

1/2 avocado, sliced

Sesame seeds

Juice of 1/2 lemon

Instructions:

1.   Start by filling the bottom of the Coconut Bowls with spinach.

2.   Place the corn, edamame, cabbage, carrots, cooked quinoa, radish, sprouts, & avocado in small piles on top of the bowls.

3.   Sprinkle with sesame seeds.

4.   Dress with some lemon juice if desired

Caramelized Banana & Blueberry Tacos

Nutritional Facts

Serving per container	7
Prep total	10 min
Serving size 2/3 cup (51g)	
Amount per serving	11
Calories	
	% Daily Value
Total Fat 2g	**2%**
Saturated Fat 7g	10%
Trans Fat 3g	8%
Cholesterol	**9%**
Sodium 470mg	**2%**
Total Carbohydrate 20g	**200%**
Dietary Fiber 10g	20%
Total Sugar 9g	1%
Protein 6g	
Vitamin C 1mcg	20%
Calcium 700mg	7%
Iron 7mg	2%
Potassium 470mg	9%

Ingredients

4 flour tortillas

1 Teaspoon coconut oil

2 ripe bananas, peeled and sliced lengthways into 0.5cm / 0.2″ slices

31

100g / 3.5oz fresh blueberries

1 Teaspoon maple syrup

3 Teaspoon vanilla favored coconut or soy yogurt

1 heaped teaspoon tahini

1.5 Teaspoon shredded coconut or coconut flakes

1 Teaspoon cacao nibs

Instructions:

1.   You will need to preheat the oven to 160°C / 320°F.

2.   Kindly wrap the tortillas in foil & heat in the oven for 6 minutes.

3.   Heat a medium-sized, heavy-based, non-stick or cast-iron skillet on medium heat on the stove. Add original coconut oil & once it's melted, add the sliced clean bananas.

4.   Fry the bananas until they are golden brown on both sides, making sure to rotate them frequently so they won't stick to the pan.

5.   You need to top the warm tortillas with the fried bananas and drizzle with tahini, yogurt, and maple syrup.

6.   Kindly top with blueberries and sprinkle with coconut and cacao nibs.

7.   Serve and enjoy

Decent Beef and Onion Stew

Serving: 4

Prep Time: 10 minutes

Cook Time 1-2 hours

Ingredients:

2 pounds lean beef, cubed

3 pounds shallots, peeled

5 garlic cloves, peeled, whole

3 tablespoons tomato paste

1 bay leaves

¼ cup olive oil

3 tablespoons lemon juice

How To:

1.   Take a stew pot and place it over medium heat.

2.   Add vegetable oil and let it heat up.

3.   Add meat and brown.

4.   Add remaining ingredients and canopy with water.

5.   Bring the entire mix to a boil.

6.   Reduce heat to low and canopy the pot.

7.   Simmer for 1-2 hours until beef is cooked thoroughly.

8.   Serve hot!

Nutrition (Per Serving)

Calories: 136

Fat: 3g

Carbohydrates: 0.9g

Protein: 24g

Clean Parsley and Chicken Breast

Serving: 2

Prep Time: 10 minutes

Cook Time: 40 minutes

Ingredients:

1/2 tablespoon dry parsley

1/2 tablespoon dry basil

2 chicken breast halves, boneless and skinless 1/4 teaspoon sunflower seeds

1/4 teaspoon red pepper flakes, crushed 1 tomato, sliced

How To:

1.   Pre-heat your oven to 350 degrees F.

2.   Take a 9x13 inch baking dish and grease it up with cooking spray.

3.   Sprinkle 1 tablespoon of parsley, 1 teaspoon of basil and spread the mixture over your baking dish.

4.   Arrange the pigeon breast halves over the dish and sprinkle garlic slices on top.

5.   Take a little bowl and add 1 teaspoon parsley, 1 teaspoon of basil, sunflower seeds, basil, red pepper and blend well. Pour the mixture over the pigeon breast.

6.   Top with tomato slices and canopy, bake for 25 minutes.

7.   Remove the duvet and bake for quarter-hour more.

8.   Serve and enjoy!

Nutrition (Per Serving)

Calories: 150

Fat: 4g

Carbohydrates: 4g

Protein: 25g

Roasted Red Pepper and Tomato Soup

Since my favorite lunch is grilled cheese sandwiches, I had to, of course, make tomato soup as a perfect match, so I thought of making it more sumptuous by adding tomatoes and red pepper and roasting them altogether. It might not be as quick as a canned tomato, but trust me, it's worth every single minute. While the soup simmers, it's easy to put the grilled cheese sandwiches together, and you'll have your desired meal.

SmartPoints value: Green plan - 1SP, Blue plan - 1SP, Purple plan - 1SP

Total Time: 1hr 20min, Prep time: 10 min, Cooking time: 1hr 10mins,

Serves: 6

Nutritional value: Calories – 107, Carbs – 19.4g, Fat – 0.4g, Protein – 4g

Ingredients

Plum tomatoes - 10 pieces

Bell peppers (red) - 3 pieces

Onion - 1 small

Olive oil - 1 tbsp

Garlic - 4 cloves

Tomato paste - 1/4 cup

Apple cider vinegar - 3 tbsp

Paprika - 1 tsp

Oregano (dried) - 1 tsp

Thyme (dried) - 1 tsp

A small handful of basil

Desired salt and pepper to taste

Instructions

1.   With a cooking spray, line a large rimmed baking sheet and put it in an over 400 degrees preheated oven.

2.   Slice each tomato into four slices, remove the seeds inside the pepper and slice into eighths. Place the peppers, garlic cloves and tomatoes onto the prepared baking sheet and mist with an olive oil mister. Evenly sprinkle the paprika, oregano, thyme, and salt and pepper on top, then place in oven and roast for 30-35 minutes.

3.   In a large pot, heat the olive oil and add diced onions and sauté and leave until they begin to soften in about 2 minutes.

4.   Lower the heat and add roasted vegetables and garlic cloves, able cider vinegar, tomato paste, fresh basil, and two cups of water. Blend using the immersion blender until it gets smooth.

5.   Lower the heat further and add in the roasted vegetables and garlic cloves, tomato paste, able cider vinegar, fresh basil, and two cups of water, add water to achieve desired consistency.

6.   Add pepper and salt to taste and cover on low heat. Stir for about 20-30 minutes regularly.

7.   This homemade meal is sure to become your gateway. Savor the flavor of the roasted veggies and garlic.

Black Bean-Tomato Chili

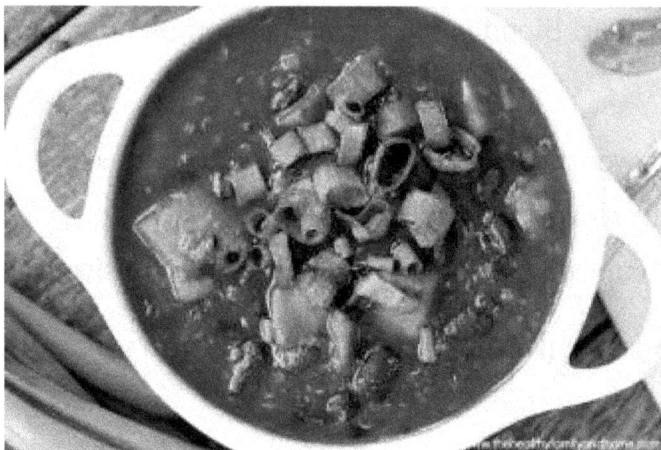

Total Time

Prep: 10 min. Cook: 35 min.

Makes

6 servings (2-1/4 quarts)

Ingredients:

2 tablespoons olive oil

1 huge onion, cleaved

1 medium green pepper, cleaved

3 garlic cloves, minced

1 teaspoon ground cinnamon

1 teaspoon ground cumin

1 teaspoon bean stew powder

1/4 teaspoon pepper

3 jars (14-1/2 ounces each) diced tomatoes, undrained

2 jars (15 ounces each) dark beans, washed and depleted

1 cup squeezed orange or juice from 3 medium oranges

Directions:

1.   In a Dutch broiler, heat oil over medium-high warmth. Include onion and green pepper; cook and mix 8-10 minutes or until delicate. Include garlic and seasonings; cook brief longer.

2.   Mix in residual fixings; heat to the point of boiling. Lessen heat; stew, secured, 20-25 minutes to enable flavors to mix, blending incidentally.

Mushroom & Broccoli Soup

Total Time

Prep: 20 min. Cook: 45 min.

Makes

8 servings

Ingredients:

1 bundle broccoli (around 1-1/2 pounds)

1 tablespoon canola oil

1/2 pound cut crisp mushrooms

1 tablespoon diminished sodium soy sauce

2 medium carrots, finely slashed

2 celery ribs, finely slashed

1/4 cup finely slashed onion

1 garlic clove, minced

1 container (32 ounces) vegetable juices

2 cups of water

2 tablespoons lemon juice

Directions:

1.   Cut broccoli florets into reduced down pieces. Strip and hack stalks.

2.   In an enormous pot, heat oil over medium-high warmth; saute mushrooms until delicate, 4-6 minutes. Mix in soy sauce; expel from skillet.

3.   In the same container, join broccoli stalks, carrots, celery, onion, garlic, soup, and water; heat to the point of boiling. Diminish heat; stew, revealed, until vegetables are relaxed, 25-30 minutes.

4.   Puree soup utilizing a drenching blender. Or then again, cool marginally and puree the soup in a blender; come back to the dish. Mix in florets and mushrooms; heat to the point of boiling. Lessen warmth to medium; cook until broccoli is delicate, 8-10 minutes, blending infrequently. Mix in lemon juice.

Avocado Fruit Salad with Tangerine Vinaigrette

Total Time

Prep/Total Time: 25 min.

Makes

8 servings

Ingredients:

3 medium ready avocados, stripped and meagerly cut

3 medium mangoes, stripped and meagerly cut

1 cup crisp raspberries

1 cup crisp blackberries

1/4 cup minced crisp mint

1/4 cup cut almonds, toasted

Dressing:

1/2 cup olive oil

1 teaspoon ground tangerine or orange strip 1/4 cup tangerine or squeezed orange

2 tablespoons balsamic vinegar

1/2 teaspoon salt

1/4 teaspoon naturally ground pepper

Directions:

1.   Mastermind avocados and organic product on a serving plate; sprinkle with mint and almonds. In a little bowl, whisk dressing fixings until mixed; shower over a plate of mixed greens.

2.   To toast nuts, prepare in a shallow container in a 350° stove for 5-10 minutes or cook in a skillet over low warmth until softly sautéed, mixing every so often.

General Salad Cauliflower

Total Time

Prep: 25 min. Cook: 20 min.

Makes

4 servings

Ingredients:

Oil for profound fat fricasseeing

1/2 cup generally useful flour

1/2 cup cornstarch

1 teaspoon salt

1 teaspoon preparing powder

3/4 cup club pop

1 medium head cauliflower, cut into 1-inch florets (around 6 cups)

Sauce:

1/4 cup squeezed orange

3 tablespoons sugar

3 tablespoons soy sauce

3 tablespoons vegetable stock

2 tablespoons rice vinegar

2 teaspoons sesame oil

2 teaspoons cornstarch

2 tablespoons canola oil

2 to 6 dried pasilla or other hot chilies, cleaved

3 green onions, white part minced, green part daintily cut

3 garlic cloves, minced

1 teaspoon ground new gingerroot

1/2 teaspoon ground orange get-up-and-go 4 cups hot cooked rice

Directions:

1.   In an electric skillet or profound fryer, heat oil to 375°. Consolidate flour, cornstarch, salt, and heating powder. Mix in club soft drink just until mixed (hitter will be slender). Plunge florets, a couple at once, into the player and fry until cauliflower are delicate and covering is light dark colored, 8-10 minutes. Channel on paper towels.

2.   For the sauce, whisk together the initial six fixings; race in cornstarch until smooth.

3.   In a huge pot, heat canola oil over medium-high warmth. Include chilies; cook and mix until fragrant, 2 minutes. Include white piece of onions, garlic, ginger, and orange get-up-and-go; cook until fragrant, around 1 moment. Mix soy sauce blend; add to the pan. Heat to the point of boiling; cook and mix until thickened, 4 minutes.

4.   Add cauliflower to sauce; hurl to cover. Present with rice; sprinkle with daintily cut green onions.

Salad Chickpea Mint Tabbouleh

Total Time

Prep/Total Time: 30 min.

Makes

4 servings

Ingredients:

1 cup bulgur

2 cups of water

1 cup new or solidified peas (around 5 ounces), defrosted

1 can (15 ounces) chickpeas or garbanzo beans, washed and depleted

1/2 cup minced new parsley

1/4 cup minced new mint

1/4 cup olive oil

2 tablespoons julienned delicate sun-dried tomatoes (not stuffed in oil)

2 tablespoons lemon juice

1/2 teaspoon salt

1/4 teaspoon pepper

Directions:

1.   In a huge pot, consolidate bulgur and water; heat to the point of boiling. Decrease heat; stew, secured, 10 minutes. Mix in crisp or solidified peas; cook, secured, until bulgur and peas are delicate, around 5 minutes.

2.   Move to an enormous bowl. Mix in outstanding fixings. Serve warm, or refrigerate and serve cold.

Creamy Cauliflower Pakora Soup

Total Time

Prep: 20 min. Cook: 20 min.

Makes

8 servings (3 quarts)

Ingredients:

1 huge head cauliflower, cut into little florets

5 medium potatoes, stripped and diced

1 huge onion, diced

4 medium carrots, stripped and diced

2 celery ribs, diced

1 container (32 ounces) vegetable stock

1 teaspoon garam masala

1 teaspoon garlic powder

1 teaspoon ground coriander

1 teaspoon ground turmeric

1 teaspoon ground cumin

1 teaspoon pepper

1 teaspoon salt

1/2 teaspoon squashed red pepper chips Water or extra vegetable stock New cilantro leaves

Lime wedges, discretionary

Directions

1.   In a Dutch stove over medium-high warmth, heat initial 14 fixings to the point of boiling. Cook and mix until vegetables are delicate, around 20 minutes. Expel from heat; cool marginally. Procedure in groups in a blender or nourishment processor until smooth. Modify consistency as wanted with water (or extra stock). Sprinkle with new cilantro. Serve hot, with lime wedges whenever wanted.

2.   Stop alternative: Before including cilantro, solidify cooled soup in cooler compartments. To utilize, in part defrost in cooler medium-term. Warmth through in a pan, blending every so often and including a little water if fundamental. Sprinkle with cilantro. Whenever wanted, present with lime wedges.

Spice Trade Beans and Bulgur

Total Time

Prep: 30 min. Cook: 3-1/2 hours

Makes

10 servings

Ingredients:

3 tablespoons canola oil, isolated

2 medium onions, slashed

1 medium sweet red pepper, slashed

5 garlic cloves, minced

1 tablespoon ground cumin

1 tablespoon paprika

2 teaspoons ground ginger

1 teaspoon pepper

1/2 teaspoon ground cinnamon

1/2 teaspoon cayenne pepper

1-1/2 cups bulgur

1 can (28 ounces) squashed tomatoes

1 can (14-1/2 ounces) diced tomatoes, undrained

1 container (32 ounces) vegetable juices

2 tablespoons darker sugar

2 tablespoons soy sauce

1 can (15 ounces) garbanzo beans or chickpeas, flushed and depleted

1/2 cup brilliant raisins

Minced crisp cilantro, discretionary

Directions:

1.   In an enormous skillet, heat 2 tablespoons oil over medium-high warmth. Include onions and pepper; cook and mix until delicate, 3-4 minutes. Include garlic and seasonings; cook brief longer. Move to a 5-qt. slow cooker.

2.   In the same skillet, heat remaining oil over medium-high warmth. Include bulgur; cook and mix until daintily caramelized, 2-3 minutes or until softly sautéed.

3.   Include bulgur, tomatoes, stock, darker sugar, and soy sauce to slow cooker. Cook, secured, on low 3-4 hours or until bulgur is delicate. Mix in beans and raisins; cook 30 minutes longer.

Whenever wanted, sprinkle with cilantro.

Tofu Chow Mein

Total Time

Prep: 15 min. + standing Cook: 15 min.

Makes

4 servings

Ingredients:

8 ounces uncooked entire wheat holy messenger hair pasta

3 tablespoons sesame oil, separated

1 bundle (16 ounces) extra-firm tofu

2 cups cut new mushrooms

1 medium sweet red pepper, julienned

1/4 cup decreased sodium soy sauce

3 green onions daintily cut

Directions:

1.   Cook pasta as per bundle headings. Channel; flush with cold water and channel once more. Hurl with 1 tablespoon oil;

spread onto a preparing sheet and let remain around 60 minutes.

2.   In the meantime, cut tofu into 1/2-in. 3D shapes and smudge dry. Enclose by a spotless kitchen towel; place on a plate and refrigerate until prepared to cook.

3.   In an enormous skillet, heat 1 tablespoon oil over medium warmth. Include pasta, spreading equitably; cook until base is daintily caramelized, around 5 minutes. Expel from skillet.

4.   In the same skillet, heat remaining oil over medium-high warmth; pan sear mushrooms, pepper, and tofu until mushrooms are delicate, 3-4 minutes. Include pasta and soy sauce; hurl and warmth through. Sprinkle with green onions.

Broiled Tilapia

SmartPoints value: Green plan - 2SP, Blue plan - 0SP, Purple plan - 0SP

Total Time: 13 min, Prep time: 8 min, Cooking time: 5 min, Serves: 4

Nutritional value: Cal - 154.8, Carbs - 1.5g, Fat - 6.4g, Protein - 22.8g

You can apply this recipe with other types of fish, such as sole, halibut, flounder, and even shellfish. You also swap lime juice for lemon juice.

Ingredients

Black pepper - ¼ tsp, freshly ground

Cooking spray - 1 spray(s)

Garlic (herb seasoning) - 2 tsp

Lemon juice (fresh) - 1 Tbsp

Table salt - ½ tsp (or to taste)

Tilapia fillet(s) (uncooked) - 20 oz, four 5 oz fillets

Instructions

1.   Prepare your grill by preheating. Coat a skillet with cooking spray.

2.   Apply seasoning to both sides of the fish with salt and pepper.

3.   Transfer the fish to the prepared skillet and drizzle it with lemon juice, then sprinkle garlic herb seasoning over the top.

4.   Broil the fish until it is fork-tender; about 5 minutes.

Grilled Miso-Glazed Cod

SmartPoints value: Green plan - 3SP, Blue plan - 2SP, Purple plan - 2SP

Total Time: 35 min, Prep time: 10 min, Cooking time: 15 min, Serves: 4

Nutritional value: Cal - 227.2, Carbs - 15.0g, Fat - 3.1g, Protein - 30.0g

This marinade produces a fantastic glaze for grilled cod. You can pair it with grilled scallions, drizzled with low-sodium soy sauce, and sesame oil to make a complete meal. If you don't have a fish basket, put foil on one area of your grill to prevent the fish from sticking out below it. Alternatively, you can broil the fish instead. Cod makes a perfect choice for grilling. Flip the fish when it starts to flake and turn opaque. Use a spatula with a broader mouth when turning the fish to help prevent the fish from breaking apart when turning. It is preferable to serve this dish with roasted carrots or broccoli.

Ingredients

White miso - 3 Tbsp

Sugar (dark brown) - 1½ Tbsp

Sake - 1 Tbsp

Mirin - ½ fl oz, (1 Tbsp)

Atlantic cod (uncooked) - 20 oz, (fillets, skin removed

Cooking spray - 1 spray(s)

Uncooked scallion(s) (chopped) - 2 Tbsp

Instructions

1.   Whisk together miso, sugar, sake, and mirin in a small bowl and spread the mixture over the cod. Cover the cod and refrigerate for at least 2 hours or up to 24 hours.

2.   Coat a grill pan off the heat with cooking spray and preheat to medium heat.

3.   Remove the cod from marinade (reserve marinade). Place it in a fish grilling basket and grill until the cod is opaque and flakes easily with a fork.

4.   Grill each side for about 5 to 7 min (brush the cod with the remaining marinade half-way through the grilling phase to create a thicker glaze). Serve the cod garnished with scallions.

Grilled Tuna with Herb Butter

SmartPoints value: Green plan - 4SP, Blue plan - 3SP, Purple plan - 3SP

Total Time: 18 min, Prep time: 12 min, Cooking time: 6 min, Serves: 4

Nutritional value: Calories - 192.0, Carbs - 8.3g, Fat - 2.5g, Protein - 38.3g

You can prepare this grilled tuna recipe in under 20 minutes. Drizzle some olive oil and lime over the tuna before you start cooking it for a unique flavor. You can nicely substitute with a lemon if you don't have a lime. I will recommend that you use salted butter for the sauce instead of unsalted butter to enhance the flavor of the dish. The secret ingredient in this grilled fish recipe is the freshly made herb butter. It also tastes great when drizzled over the spinach.

Ingredients

Olive oil - 1 tsp

Lime juice (fresh) - 1 tsp

Black pepper - ⅛ tsp, or to taste

Cooking spray - 1 spray(s)

Salted butter - 2 Tbsp, softened

Chives (finely chopped) - 1 Tbsp, fresh

Parsley (fresh) - 1 Tbsp, finely chopped

Tarragon (fresh) - 1 Tbsp, finely chopped

Lime zest (fresh, minced) - 1 tsp

Table salt - ¼ tsp, or to taste

Spinach (fresh) - 1 pound(s), baby-variety, steamed

Yellowfin tuna (uncooked) - 1 pound(s), one steak cut 1- to 1-1/2 inches thick

Instructions

1.   Drizzle oil and lime juice on both sides of the fish and set it aside.

2.   Coat your grill with cooking spray off heat, and preheat the grill on high heat.

3.   Combine softened butter, chives, parsley, tarragon, lime zest, salt, and pepper in a small metal bowl and then set aside.

4.   Grill the tuna on one side for three minutes, then carefully turn it and cook on the other side for another three minutes or longer until you have achieved the desired degree of cooking.

5.   Place the bowl containing butter mixture on the grill just until it melts. Don't let it cook.

6.   Slice the tuna thinly and serve it over spinach, then drizzle melted herb butter over the top.

Notes: If you prefer, you can broil the tuna on a grill pan. In this recipe, you will prepare the tuna like a steak. In case you prefer your tuna to be more well done, add about 1 minute to your total cooking time. However, tuna cooks rapidly, so make sure you do not overcook it. The herb butter is excellent on both the tuna and the spinach.

Lemon-Herb Roasted Salmon

SmartPoints value: Green plan - 5SP, Blue plan - 2SP, Purple plan - 2SP

Total Time: 31 min, Prep time: 16 min, Cooking time: 15 min, Serves: 4

Nutritional value: Calories - 118.1, Carbs - 1.0g, Fat - 6.8g, Protein - 12.9g

Give your family a fabulous salmon flavor with lemon juice, lemon zest, and fresh herbs in this easy entrée that will be ready in about 30 minutes. I have used pink salmon fillets because they are less fatty compared to some other salmon varieties like sockeye and Coho salmon.

The salmon should flake when pierced with a fork. That's an excellent indicator that it is ready. Ensure that you zest the lemon before juicing it.

To produce enough zest and juice for this recipe, you will need about two lemons. The mix of fresh herbs in this dish is lovely. However, you can use whatever combination you like; this recipe is versatile. Stir a few red pepper flakes into the herb mixture to add a little heat.

Ingredients

Black pepper (coarsely ground) - ⅛ tsp (or to taste)

Cooking spray - 1 spray(s)

Lemon juice (fresh) - 4 Tbsp, divided

Lemon zest (finely grated) - 1 tsp (with extra for garnish, if you like)

Minced garlic - 1 tsp

Oregano (fresh) - 1 tsp

Parsley (fresh, chopped) - 1 Tbsp (with extra for garnish, if you like)

Uncooked wild pink salmon fillet(s) (also known as humpback salmon) - 1½ pound(s), four 6-oz pieces about 1-inch-thick each

Table salt - ⅛ tsp (or to taste)

Sugar - 1½ Tbsp

Thyme (fresh, chopped) - 1 Tbsp (with extra for garnish, if you like)

Instructions

1.   Heat your oven to 400°F before using it. Get a small, shallow baking dish and coat it with cooking spray.

2.   Apply seasoning to both sides of the salmon with salt and pepper, then place the salmon in the prepared baking dish and drizzle on it with two tablespoons of lemon juice.

3.   Whisk the remaining two tablespoons of lemon juice, sugar, parsley, thyme, lemon zest, garlic, and oregano together in a small bowl, then continue whisking until the sugar dissolves in the mixture and set it aside.

4.   Roast the salmon until it is close to being ready; about 13 minutes, then remove it from the oven and top it with the lemon-herb mixture.

5.   Return it to the oven and allow it to roast until the salmon is fork-tender, about 2 minutes more. Garnish the dish with fresh herbs that you chopped and the grated zest, if you like.

Grilled Tuna Provencal

SmartPoints value: Green plan - 3SP, Blue plan - 2SP, Purple plan - 2SP

Total Time: 20 min, Prep time: 10 min, Cooking time: 10 min, Serves: 4

Nutritional value: Calories - 335, Carbs - 14.6g, Fat - 15.5g, Protein - 36.1g

This one-dish meal is usually ready in just 20 minutes, oozing with a delicious French flavor. You can make the whole meal in one pan, aiding clean up after cooking. To cook with a grill pan and get the best result, you need to preheat the pan for at least five minutes to ensure that you distribute the heat evenly. That will help you avoid overcooking parts of the meat while not cooking other parts. If you're not sure about the hotness of the grill pan, drop a half teaspoon of water on there to see if it evaporates.

With steamed spinach or a bed of rice, this dish tastes lovely.

Ingredients

Black pepper (freshly ground, divided) - ¾ tsp

Cooking spray - 3 spray(s)

Uncooked tuna (about 1- to 1 1/2-in thick) - 1 pound(s)

Olive(s) (pitted and chopped)- 6 large

Olive oil - 1 Tbsp

Rosemary (fresh, minced) - 1 Tbsp

Red wine - 2 fl oz

Sea salt - ¾ tsp, divided

Tomato(es) (fresh, diced) - 2½ cup(s)

Garlic clove(s) (minced) - 2 medium clove(s)

Parsley (fresh, minced) - 2 Tbsp

Sugar - ⅛ tsp

Instructions

1.   Wash the tuna thoroughly and pat it dry. Rub 1/4 teaspoon each of salt and pepper over it, then set it aside.

2.   Combine tomatoes, parsley, rosemary, garlic, olives, oil, and the remaining 1/2 teaspoon each of salt and pepper in a separate bowl, then set it aside.

3.   Get a reasonably large grill pan and coat it with cooking spray, then set it over medium-high heat. When the pan is visibly hot, cook the tuna for 2 to 3 minutes (or longer) per side for a rare cook (or thorough cook). As soon as you have prepared

the tuna, remove it to a serving plate and wrap it with aluminum foil to keep it warm.

4.	Add the red wine, tomato mixture, and sugar to the hot grill pan and cook, scraping the bottom of the pan frequently, until the tomato mixture reduces to about two cups. The alcohol must have cooked off.

5.	Remove foil from the tuna, slice it thinly, and serve with tomato mixture over the top.

Southern-Style Oven-Fried Chicken

SmartPoints value: Green plan - 4SP, Blue Plan - 3SP, Purple plan - 3SP

Total Time: 45 min, Prep time: 15 min, Cooking time: 30 min, Serves: 4

Nutritional value: Calories - 256.9, Carbs - 31.3g, Fat - 1.6g, Protein - 27.5g

Switch to oven frying and lighten up this favorite hearty dish. I decided to improve the flavor by adding buttermilk and a pinch of cayenne pepper.

Ingredients

All-purpose flour - ⅓ cup(s)

Buttermilk (low-fat) - 3 oz

Cayenne pepper - ¼ tsp (or to taste), divided

Cooking spray - 3 spray(s)

Cornflake crumbs - ½ cup(s)

Table salt - ½ tsp (or to taste), divided

Uncooked chicken breast(s) - 1 pound(s), four 4-oz pieces (boneless, skinless)

Instructions

1.   Heat the oven to 375°F before starting. Coat a 13- X 8- X 2-inch baking dish lightly with cooking spray and set it aside.

2.   Add salt and cayenne pepper to chicken for a tasty seasoning and set it aside also.

3.   Put a mixture of flour, 1/4 teaspoon salt, and 1/8 teaspoon cayenne pepper in a bowl of medium size.

4.   Put the buttermilk and cornflakes crumbs in 2 separate shallow bowls.

5.   Dip the chicken in the flour mixture and evenly coat both sides.

6.   Next, dip the flour-coated chicken into buttermilk and turn it to coat both sides.

7.   Finally, dip the coated chicken in cornflake crumbs and turn to coat both sides.

8.   Place coated chicken breasts in the baking dish that you prepared.

9.   Bake the chicken until it is tender and no longer pink in the center (you don't need to flip the chicken while baking). The baking should take about 25 to 30 minutes.

Italian Chicken Soup with Vegetables

SmartPoints value: Green plan - 4SP, Blue plan - 1SP, Purple plan - 1SP

Total Time: 27 min, Prep time: 15 min, Cooking time: 12 min, Serves: 1

Nutritional value: Calories - 136.7, Carbs - 22.3g, Fat - 1.0g, Protein - 9.6g

This chicken soup is ideal for a leisurely lunch or a quick dinner, as it is brothy and filled with vegetables. To make it bulky, you can add in any cooked grain you have on hand, like rice, barley, or quinoa, which will also add some nice texture and make it more chewable. You can use any leftover chicken you have. The drizzle of extra virgin olive oil at the end not only makes the soup look a little fancier, but it can also add a rich flavor that takes a simple soup like this one to the next level.

Ingredients

Chicken broth - 1 cup(s), canned

Chicken breast(s) - 1 cup(s), diced (skinless, boneless)

Extra virgin olive oil - 1 tsp, divided

Fresh thyme - 1¼ tsp (leaves)

Fresh mushroom(s) - 1 cup(s), sliced

Garlic clove(s) - 1 medium-sized, minced

Green beans - 1 small bowl, cooked

Lemon(s) - 1 slice(s)

Plum tomato(es) - 1 medium-sized, diced

Uncooked cauliflower - 1 cup(s), small florets

Instructions

1.   Heat 1/2 tsp of olive oil in a small skillet over medium heat.

2.   Add the mushrooms and garlic, then cook, continuously stirring until mushrooms begin to soften and the mixture is fragrant; about 2 minutes.

3.   Add the broth in the chicken and bring it to a boil over medium-high heat.

4.   Add cauliflower and (or) green beans, then reduce the heat to medium-low and simmer until it is almost tender; about 4 minutes.

5.   Add the chicken, thyme, and tomatoes, then simmer until the vegetables are tender; about 2 minutes.

6.   Drizzle it with the remaining 1/2 tsp of oil and fresh lemon juice, then grind the pepper over the top, if you desire.

Roasted Chicken Breast with Spiced Cauliflower

SmartPoints value: Green plan - 4SP, Blue plan - 2SP, Purple plan - 2SP

Total Time: 50 min, Prep time: 20 min, Cooking time: 30 min, Serves: 4

Nutritional value: Calories - 470.9, Carbs - 3.5g, Fat - 11.3g, Protein - 84.2g

In this tasty recipe, you will brush chicken breasts with olive oil, turmeric, ground coriander, and cumin, with a touch of cayenne pepper before roasting, and surround it by a bed of cauliflower florets.

After cooking the chicken thoroughly, toss the cauliflower in all the delicious juices in the skillet, and let it continue to roast until it's sweet and tender. You can't have anything more convenient than a single-sheet pan dinner on a busy weeknight.

Drizzle fresh lime juice and sprinkle fresh cilantro into this Indian-influenced meal to add incredible flavor. In case you don't like cilantro, parsley or oregano works well too.

Ingredients

Black pepper (divided) - ½ tsp

Cayenne pepper - ⅛ tsp

Cooking spray - 2 spray(s)

Cilantro (finely chopped) - 1 Tbsp

Olive oil - 2 Tbsp

Coriander (ground) - 1 tsp

Turmeric (ground) - 1 tsp

Durkee Cumin (ground) - ½ tsp

Kosher salt (divided) - ¾ tsp

Uncooked chicken breast - 1 pound(s), two 8 oz pieces (boneless, skinless)

Uncooked cauliflower - 1 pound(s), cut into bite-size pieces

Fresh lime(s) - ½ medium, with wedges for serving

Instructions

1.   Before you start, heat the oven to 450°F. Get a large baking sheet and line it with parchment paper.

2.   Combine and mix oil, turmeric, coriander, cumin, 1/2 tsp of salt, 1/4 tsp of pepper, and cayenne in a large bowl.

3.   Place the chicken in the center of the prepared baking sheet and brush each piece with 1/2 tsp of oil mixture.

4.   Add cauliflower to the bowl and toss it to coat. Place the cauliflower around the chicken and lightly coat both chicken and cauliflower with cooking spray.

5.   Sprinkle the chicken with the remaining 1/4 tsp of each salt and pepper.

6.   Roast the coated chicken until it cooks through; 15-20 minutes and let it rest.

7.   Toss the cauliflower and chicken juices in the pan, then continue roasting until browned and tender; about 10 minutes more.

8.   Add the cilantro and toss again.

9.   Thickly slice the chicken across the grain and fan over serving plates.

10.   Serve the cauliflower and chicken in each plate and squeeze 1/2 lime over the top, then serve with additional lime wedges.

Vietnamese Chicken and Veggie Bowl with Rice Noodles

SmartPoints value: Green plan - 6SP, Blue plan - 4SP, Purple plan - 4SP

Total Time: 26 min, Prep time: 20 min, Cooking time: 6 min, Serves: 1

Nutritional value: Calories - 280.4, Carbs - 42.3g, Fat - 10.0g, Protein - 9.1g

This dish is a delicious and stunning entrée that comes together in just 25 minutes. It is a perfect recipe for one. You can even use leftover cooked chicken breast and grilled vegetables.

I would prefer you to use chicken cutlets with broccoli and red peppers, but feel free to experiment with chicken thighs, spinach, mushrooms, onions, or whatever you have on hand.

The soy and fish sauces add that ultimate umami bomb, while sriracha helps keep it balanced out by providing a touch of heat.

You can quickly scale up this recipe if you need to serve it to a crowd.

Ingredients

Cilantro (chopped, fresh leaves) - 2 Tbsp

Cooked rice noodles - ½ cup(s)

Asian fish sauce - ½ tsp

Cooking spray - 4 spray(s)

Uncooked chicken breast - 5 oz, thin cutlet (boneless, skinless)

Uncooked broccoli - 1 cup(s), small florets or baby stalks

Red pepper(s) (sweet) - ½ medium, cut in 2 even pieces

Soy sauce (low sodium) - 2 Tbsp, divided (or to taste)

Sriracha sauce - 1 tsp (or to taste)

Sugar - ¼ tsp

Roasted peanuts (unsalted dry) - 2 tsp, chopped

Instructions

1.   Coat a grill or grill pan with cooking spray and preheat on medium-high heat.

2.   Place the chicken, broccoli, and red pepper in a shallow bowl and drizzle with one tablespoon of soy sauce, then toss to coat.

3.   Coat the chicken with cooking spray and grill, turning the chicken once and the vegetables a few times, until chicken cooks through and veggies are tender-crisp; about 6 minutes.

4.   Slice the chicken and pepper them into strips, then place all in a bowl over noodles.

5.   Stir together the remaining one tablespoon of soy sauce, fish sauce, and sugar. Drizzle the mixture over your cooked chicken.

Sprinkle a mixture of cilantro, peanuts, and sriracha on the chicken, then serve.

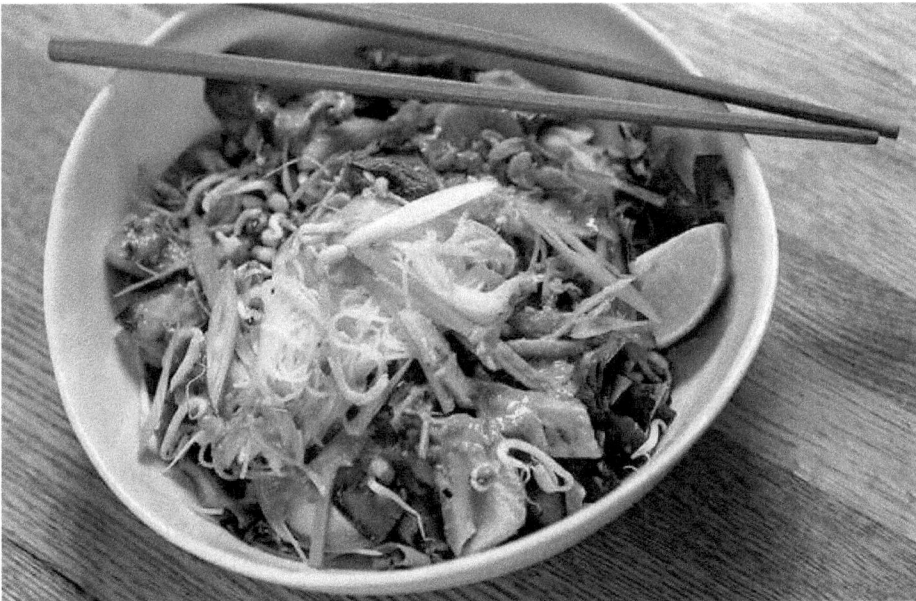

Fall Harvest Salad

SmartPoints value: Green plan - 3SP, Blue plan - 1SP, Purple plan - 1SP

Total time: 15 min, Prep time: 15 min, Cooking time: 0 min, Serves: 4

Nutritional value: Calories - 175, Carbs – 25.7g, Fat – 7.6g, Protein – 4.8g

Whether or not you have planned for a holiday meal, this fall harvest salad will fire up some inspiration, and get those juices flowing.

If this would be your first time giving this a try, I trust you'll be looking for excuses to make this salad over and over again.

There are two most seen together in desserts, that's the flavor combination of cinnamon and apples. They both make undeniable mouthwatering delicious flavors in this fall harvest salad.

I also love to add some Honey crisp apples (my favorite apple), or sometimes I use Fuji, a pink lady on this Harvest Salad. They all blend well.

To prevent my apples from getting brown after slicing, I avoid exposing it to air. When the apples turn brown, your salad would not be as pretty as you would love it. I will add a little, so that will help you avoid this problem and keep your apples beautiful

After slicing your apple, submerge the slices in a bowl of saltwater (I usually mix about 1 tbsp of salt with 1 ½ cups of water) then stir it until the salt dissolves then add in the apple slices. Let it sit for about 5 minutes and then rinse the slices with water and pat dry with a paper towel.

That's just it. So simple, yeah? This way of cutting apples has been working for me for ages, and I love it more because it's cheaper and cleaner than buying those bags of pre-cut apples.

Ingredients

Kale greens (baby variety) - 4-5 cups

Large apple (thinly sliced) - 1 piece

Sweet pumpkin seeds (toasted) - 1/3 cup

For dressing

Olive oil - 1 tbsp

Maple Syrup - 1 tbsp

Red wine vinegar - 2 tbsp

Shallot (minced) - 1 piece

Cinnamon - ¼ tsp

Dijon mustard - 1 tsp

Pepper and salt to taste

Instructions

1.   Beat all the ingredients for the dressing together in a small bowl

2.   Toss the ingredients for the salad in a large bowl

3.   Pour the processed dressing over the salad and toss to coat evenly

4.   This perfect dish is sure to impress your guests and compliment your holiday meal. Be careful not to lick the bowl.

Mediterranean Baked Tilapia

SmartPoints value: Green plan - 3SP, Blue plan - 1SP, Purple plan - 1SP

Total time: 25 min, Prep time: 10 min, Cooking time: 15 min, Serves: 4

Nutritional value: Calories - 129, Fat - 5g, Protein - 21g

During festive periods, it gets more tempting to eat just every meal that crosses by you. That's why I'm creating this recipe to help you maintain low SP meals during those periods. Let's take a look at the deliciously outlined recipe.

Ingredients

Tilapia fillets - 1 lb (about eight fillets)

Olive oil - 1 tsp

Butter - 1 tbsp

Shallots (finely chopped) - 2 pieces

Garlic (minced) - 3 cloves

Cumin (ground) - 1 1/2 tsp

Paprika (1 1/2 tsp)

Capers (1/4 cup)

Dill (finely chopped, fresh) - 1/4 cup

Lemon juice - from 1 lemon

Pepper and salt to taste

Instructions

1.   Line a rimmed baking sheet with parchment paper or foil over a preheated oven of 375 degrees. Mist with cooking spray and spread fish fillets evenly on the baking sheet.

2.   Combine the paprika, pepper, and salt in a small bowl. Season the fish fillets with the spice mixture on both sides.

3.   Whisk together in a small bowl, the melted butter, olive oil, lemon juice, shallots, and garlic then brush evenly over the fish fillets.

Top with the capers.

4.   Making sure not to overcook, bake in the oven for about 10-15 minutes, then remove from oven and top with fresh dill.

Two-Ingredient Ice Cream Cupcake Bites

SmartPoints value: Green plan - 2SP, Blue plan - 2SP, Purple plan - 2SP

Total Time: 32 min, Prep time: 5 min, Cooking time: 12 min, Serves: 12

Nutritional value: Calories - 109, Carbs - 10g, Fat - 8g, Protein - 12g

You won't get any fresh-baked dessert or snack that is easier or more lovely than these two-ingredient mini cupcakes. All it takes is to mash your favorite

WW ice cream bars and combine with self-rising flour, then bake it. You can eat it as it is or finish it off with whipped topping and sprinkles. They are perfect for birthday parties, snacks, and more.

Ingredients

Ice cream bars (WW Dark Chocolate-raspberry) - 6 bar(s) White flour (self-rising) - 10 Tbsp Whipped topping (light) - 4 Tbsp Sprinkles (rainbow) - ½ Tbsp

Instructions

1.   After preheating the oven to 350°F, coat twelve mini muffin holes with cooking spray

2.   Drop the ice cream from the sticks into a large bowl and allow it to melt slightly, then add some white flour and stir until it is well-mixed.

3.   Evenly fill prepared muffin holes with the mixture and bake until a tester inserted in the center of a cupcake comes out without anything sticking to it; about 10-12 minutes.

4.   Allow the cupcakes to cool in the pan for a few minutes before taking them out. Collect the processed muffins from the pan and cool completely.

5.   Put one teaspoon of whipped topping in each cooled cupcake and divide the sprinkles over the top.

Lemon Blueberry Cheesecake Yogurt Bark

SmartPoints value: 1SP

Total time: 1 hr 15 mins, Prep time: 15 mins, Chill time: 1 hr, Serves - 12

Nutritional value: Calories - 124, Carbs - 12.7g, Fat - 0.2g, Protein - 18.2g

Ingredients

Greek yogurt (plain non-fat) - 1 cup

Agave nectar - 1 tablespoon

Lemon zest - 1/2 teaspoon

Lemon juice (fresh-squeezed) - 1/2 teaspoon Blueberries (fresh) - 1 cup

Graham crackers (crushed into crumbs) - 3 squares (gluten-free if you like)

Instructions

1.   Line a 9x5-inch loaf pan with aluminum foil so that the foil hangs over sides of the pan.

2.   Mix the yogurt, lemon zest, agave nectar, and lemon juice in a small mixing bowl, then stir.

3.   Turn in the blueberries gently with three tablespoons crushed graham cracker crumbs just until adequately mixed.

4.   Evenly spread the mixture into the loaf pan you earlier prepared. Get the remaining cracker crumbs and sprinkle over the top.

5.   Use aluminum foil to cover the loaf pan and refrigerate for at least 1 hour; until it is frozen.

6.   Once the mixture is frozen, remove the pan from the freezer and use overhanging foil as handles to lift the bark from the pan.

7.   Put the frozen mixture on a cutting board and slice it into eight squares.

8.   Cut each square diagonally, creating two triangles. (If the frozen dough is too difficult to cut, allow it to sit out at room temperature to soften. Alternatively, you can keep the knife inside hot water before cutting.)

9.   Keep the cut portions in an airtight container inside the freezer until you are ready to serve. Allow the cut triangles to sit on the

table at room temperature to soften slightly before serving if it is too frozen.

Dark Chocolate Avocado Mousse

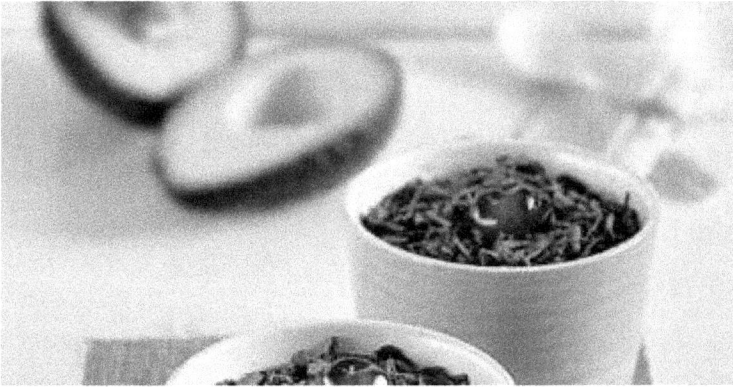

This chocolate delicacy, loaded with healthy fats, fiber, and antioxidants, is a perfect dessert recipe.

SmartPoints value - 9SP

Total time: 1 hr 10 mins, Prep time: 10 mins, Chill time: 1 hr, Serves: 2

Nutritional value: Calories - 434, Carbs - 53g, Fat - 29g, Protein - 6g

Ingredients

Avocado (very ripe, peeled and seeded) - 1 large

Dark baking chocolate (70% cacao, melted) - 2 ounces

Cocoa powder (unsweetened) - 2 Tbsp

Almond milk (unsweetened) - 1/4 cup

Maple syrup - 2 Tbsp

Pure vanilla extract - 1/4 Tsp

Cinnamon (ground) - A pinch

Salt - A pinch

Instructions

1.   Get a blender and put in avocado, maple syrup, melted chocolate, milk, cocoa powder, vanilla, cinnamon, and salt.

2.   Process the content of the blender until you get a smooth and creamy mixture. To make the mousse thinner, add more milk or less milk for a thicker mousse.

3.   Pour the mixture evenly into two small dessert glasses.

4.   Chill it for at least 1 hour in the refrigerator before serving.

Hearty Chia and Blackberry Pudding

Serving: 2

Prep Time: 45 minutes

Cook Time: Nil

Ingredients:

¼ cup chia seeds

½ cup blackberries, fresh

1 teaspoon liquid sweetener

1 cup coconut almond milk, full fat and unsweetened

1 teaspoon vanilla extract

How To:

1.   Take the vanilla, liquid sweetener and coconut almond milk and add to blender.

2.   Process until thick.

3.   Add in blackberries and process until smooth.

4.   Divide the mixture between cups and chill for 30 minutes.

5.   Serve and enjoy!

Nutrition (Per Serving)

Calories: 437

Fat: 38g

Carbohydrates: 8g

Protein: 8g

Special Cocoa Brownie Bombs

Serving: 12

Prep Time: 15 minutes

Cooking Time: 25 minutes

Freeze Time: None

Ingredients:

2 tablespoons grass-fed almond butter

1 whole egg

2 teaspoons vanilla extract

¼ teaspoon baking powder

1/3 cup heavy cream

3/4 cup almond butter

¼ cocoa powder

A pinch of sunflower seeds

How To:

1.   Break the eggs and whisk until smooth.

2.   Add in all the wet ingredients and mix well.

3.   Make the batter by mixing all the dry ingredients and sifting them into the wet ingredients.

4.   Pour into a greased baking pan.

5.   Bake for 25 minutes at 350 degrees F or until a toothpick inserted in the middle comes out clean.

6.   Let it cool, slice and serve.

Nutrition (Per Serving)

Total Carbs: 1g

Fiber: 0g

Protein: 1g

Fat: 20g

Elegant Mango Compote

Serving: 4

Prep Time: 10 minutes

Cook Time: 10 minutes

Ingredients:

4 cups mango, peeled and cubed

1 cup orange juice

6 tablespoons palm sugar

3 tablespoons lime juice

How To:

1.   Add mango, lime juice, orange juice, sugar to your Instant Pot.

2.   Lock the lid and cook on LOW pressure for 10 minutes.

3.   Release the pressure naturally over 10 minutes.

4.   Remove the lid and divide amongst serving bowls.

5.   Enjoy!

Nutrition (Per Serving)

Calories: 180

Fat: 2g

Carbohydrates: 12g

Protein: 2g

Lovely <u>Carrot</u> Cake

Prep Time: 3 hours 15 minutes

Cooking Time: Ni

Serving: 6

Ingredients:

For Cashew Frosting

2 tablespoons lemon juice

2 cups cashews, soaked

2 tablespoons coconut oil, melted 1/3 cup maple syrup water

For Cake

1 cup pineapple, dried and chopped

2 carrots, chopped

1 ½ cups coconut flour

1 cup dates, pitted

½ cup dry coconut

½ teaspoon cinnamon

How To:

1.   Add cashews, lemon juice, maple syrup, coconut oil, apple and pulse well.

2.   Transfer to a bowl and keep it on the side.

3.   Add carrots to your processor and pulse a few times.

4.   Add flour, dates, pineapple, coconut, cinnamon and pulse.

5.   Pour half of the mixture into a spring form pan and spread well.

6.   Add 1/3 of the cashew frosting and spread evenly.

7.   Add remaining cake batter and spread the frosting.

8.   Place in your freezer until it is hard.

9.   Cut and serve.

10.   Enjoy!

Nutrition (Per Serving)

Calories: 140

Fat: 4g

Carbohydrates: 8g

Protein: 4g

Grilled Peach with Honey Yogurt Dressing

Prep Time: 10 minutes

Cooking Time: 5 minutes

Serving: 6

Ingredients:

2 large peaches, ripe and halved

2 tablespoons honey

1/8 teaspoon cinnamon

¼ cut vanilla Greek yogurt, fat free

How To:

1.   Prepare your outdoor grill and heat on low heat.
2.   Grill your peaches on indirect heat until they are tender, it should take about 2-4 minutes each side.
3.   Take a bowl and mix in yogurt and cinnamon.
4.   Drizzle honey mix on top and enjoy!

Nutrition (Per Serving)
Calories: 140

Fat: 4g

Carbohydrates: 8g

Protein: 4g

Hearty Carrot Cookies

Prep Time: 10 minutes

Cooking Time: 15 minutes

Serving: 6

Ingredients:

½ cup packed light brown sugar

½ cup sugar

½ cup oil

½ cup apple sauce

2 whole eggs

1 cup flour

1 teaspoon vanilla

1 teaspoon baking soda

1 cup whole wheat flour

¼ teaspoon salt

½ teaspoon ground nutmeg

1 teaspoon cinnamon, ground

1 ½ cups carrots, grated

1 cup golden raisin

2 cups rolled oats, raw

How To:

1.   Pre-heat your oven to about 350 degrees F.

2.   Take a bowl and mix in applesauce, oil, sugar, vanilla and eggs.

3.   Take another bowl and mix in the dry ingredients.

4.   Blend the dry ingredients into the bowl with wet mixture.

5.   Stir in carrots and raisins to the mix.

6.   Take a greased cookie sheet and drop in the mixture spoon by spoon.

7.   Transfer to oven and bake for 15 minutes until you have a golden-brown texture.

8.   Serve and enjoy!

Nutrition (Per Serving)

Calories: 140

Fat: 4g

Carbohydrates: 8g

Protein: 4g

Milky Pudding

Prep Time: 10 minutes

Cooking Time: 5-10 minutes + chill time

Serving: 6

Ingredients:

3 tablespoons cornstarch

½ teaspoon vanilla

1/3 cup chocolate chips

2 cups non-fat milk

1/8 teaspoon salt

2 tablespoons salt

2 tablespoons sugar

How To:

1. Take a medium sized bowl and add cocoa powder, cornstarch, salt, sugar and mix well.

2. Whisk in the milk.

3.   Place over medium heat and keep heating until thick and bubbly.

4.   Remove the mixture from heat and stir in vanilla and chocolate chips.

5.   Keep mixing until the chips are melted and you have a smooth pudding.

6.   Pour into a large sized dish and let it chill.

7.   Serve and enjoy!

Nutrition:

Calories: 140

Fat: 4g

Carbohydrates: 8g

Protein: 4g

Fresh Honey Strawberries with Yogurt

Prep Time: 10 minutes

Cooking Time: 5-10 minutes + chill time

Serving: 6

Ingredients:

4 tablespoons almond, sliced and toasted

3 cups yogurt, low fat

4 teaspoons honey

1-pint fresh strawberries

How To:

1.   Take your strawberries and wash under water, clean well.

2.   Cut into quarters.

3.   Take your serving dishes and add ¾ cup yogurt into each dish.

4.   Divide strawberries among the dishes.

5.   Top each dish with honey, sliced almonds.

6.   Serve and enjoy!

Nutrition:

Calories: 140

Fat: 4g

Carbohydrates: 8g

Protein: 4g

Spinach Dip

Serving: 2

Prep Time: 4 minutes

Cook Time: 0 minutes

Ingredients:

5 ounces Spinach, raw

1 cup Greek yogurt

1/2 tablespoon onion powder

1/4 teaspoon garlic sunflower seeds

Black pepper to taste

1/4 teaspoon Greek Seasoning

How To:

1.	Add the listed ingredients in a blender.

2.	Emulsify.

3.	Season and serve.

Nutrition (Per Serving)

Calories: 101

Fat: 4g

Carbohydrates: 4g

Protein: 10g

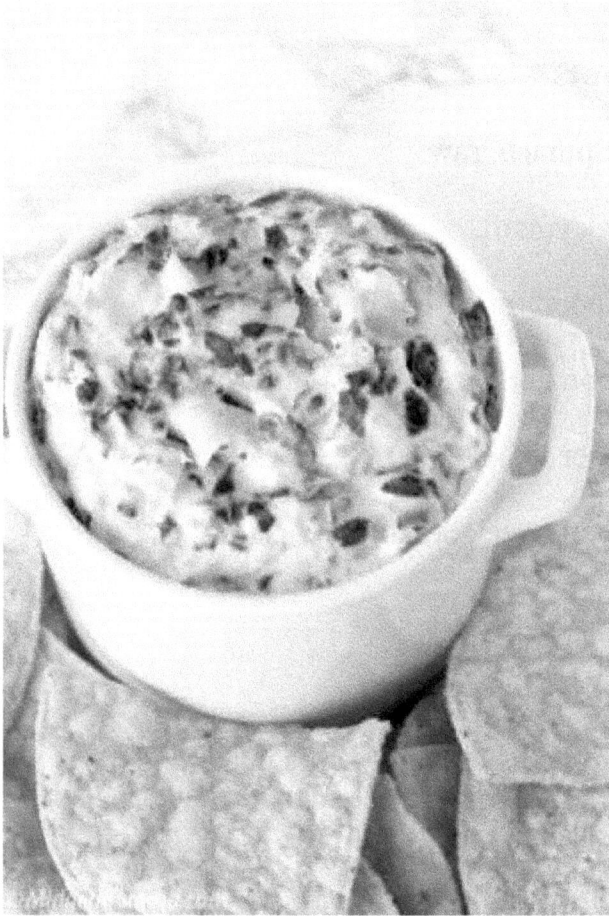

Cauliflower Rice

Serving: 2

Prep Time: 5 minutes

Cook Time: 6 minutes

Ingredients:

1 head grated cauliflower head

1 tablespoon coconut aminos

1 pinch of sunflower seeds

1 pinch of black pepper

1 tablespoon Garlic Powder

1 tablespoon Sesame Oil

How To:

1.   Add cauliflower to a food processor and grate it.

2.   Take a pan and add sesame oil, let it heat up over medium heat.

3.   Add grated cauliflower and pour coconut aminos.

4. Cook for 4-6 minutes.

5. Season and enjoy!

Nutrition (Per Serving)

Calories: 329

Fat: 28g

Carbohydrates: 13g

Protein: 10g

Grilled Sprouts and Balsamic Glaze

Serving: 2

Prep Time: 10 minutes

Cook Time: 30 minutes

Ingredients:

½ pound Brussels sprouts, trimmed and halved Fresh cracked black pepper 1 tablespoon olive oil

Sunflower seeds to taste

2 teaspoons balsamic glaze

2 wooden skewers

How To:

1.   Take wooden skewers and place them on a largely sized foil.

2.   Place sprouts on the skewers and drizzle oil, sprinkle sunflower seeds and pepper.

3.   Cover skewers with foil.

4.   Pre-heat your grill to low and place skewers (with foil) in the grill.

5.   Grill for 30 minutes, making sure to turn after every 5-6 minutes.

6.   Once done, uncovered and drizzle balsamic glaze on top.

7.   Enjoy!

Nutrition (Per Serving)

Calories: 440

Fat: 27g

Carbohydrates: 33g

Protein: 26g

Amazing Green Creamy Cabbage

Serving: 4

Prep Time: 10 minutes

Cook Time: 10 minutes

Ingredients:

2 ounces almond butter

1 ½ pounds green cabbage, shredded

1 ¼ cups coconut cream

Sunflower seeds and pepper to taste

8 tablespoons fresh parsley, chopped

How To:

1.   Take a skillet and place it over medium heat, add almond butter and let it melt.

2.   Add cabbage and sauté until brown.

3.   Stir in cream and lower the heat to low.

4.   Let it simmer.

5.   Season with sunflower seeds and pepper.

6.   Garnish with parsley and serve.

7.   Enjoy!

Nutrition (Per Serving)

Calories: 432

Fat: 42g

Carbohydrates: 8g

Protein: 4g

www.ingramcontent.com/pod-product-compliance
Lightning Source LLC
Chambersburg PA
CBHW050749030426
42336CB00012B/1724